Simplified Solution Approach

To CHRONIC

HEADACHES

Headache-Free Living: Empower Yourself with Proven Remedies from the Ultimate Guide

Dr QUENTIN GLYN

Table Of Contents

CHAPTER ONE

Chronic Headaches

A large percentage of people worldwide suffer from chronic headaches, a common and often incapacitating medical disease. The everyday functioning, productivity, and general well-being of a person may all be greatly impacted by these chronic and recurrent headaches.

We will explore the idea of chronic headaches in this talk, giving a thorough explanation, characterizing the many kinds, looking at how they affect quality of life, and looking at common causes and triggers.

An Overview Of Prolonged Headaches

A chronic headache is defined as ongoing, recurrent headache pain that lasts for at least three months and occurs on 15 or more days per month. Chronic headaches may become a persistent and difficult part of everyday life, in contrast to episodic headaches, which are rare and transient. The disorder includes a range of headache kinds, each with distinct traits, symptoms, and methods of therapy.

Types And Definitions:

Definition: Long-lasting, persistent headaches that interfere with everyday activities and quality of life may be generally referred to as chronic headaches.

Differentiating between primary and secondary chronic headaches is important. Secondary chronic headaches are signs of various underlying medical diseases, while primary chronic headaches—such as cluster headaches, tension-type headaches, and chronic migraines—are illnesses unto themselves.

Chronic Headache Types:

Recurrent moderate to severe headaches, often accompanied by nausea, vomiting, and light and sound sensitivity, are the hallmarks of chronic migraine.

Persistent Tension-Type Headache: Consists of a tightening, pressing, or pressing feeling around the head, often accompanied by tension in the shoulders and neck muscles.

Chronic Cluster Headache: Characterized by acute, unilateral pain in the area around the eye or temple, interspersed with intervals without headaches and extreme pain episodes called clusters.

Hemicrania Continua: An uncommon kind of headache characterized by constant, ongoing discomfort on one side of the head or face.

New Daily Persistent Headache (NDPH): Usually has tightness or pressing sensation, it starts off abruptly and lasts all day.

For successful management and treatment of persistent headaches, it is essential to identify the particular kind of headache.

Effect On Life Quality:

Persistent headaches may significantly lower a person's quality of life. When paired with other symptoms like light sensitivity and nausea, the chronic pain might result in:

Reduced Work Performance: Prolonged headaches may impair focus, output, and general job performance.

Social and Recreational Restrictions: People who suffer from chronic headaches may steer clear of social gatherings and leisure pursuits out of concern that they would aggravate or start their headaches.

Effects on Emotional and Mental Health: Prolonged suffering and disruptions to regular life may cause anxiety, sadness, and emotional discomfort.

Reduced Sleep Quality: People who have chronic headaches often have sleep difficulties, which adds to the overall negative effect on well-being.

Typical Causes And Initiators:

Identifying the triggers and underlying causes of persistent headaches is essential to creating successful treatment plans. Typical elements consist of:

Genetic Predisposition: Certain people may be more prone to persistent headaches due to a genetic predisposition.

Environmental elements: Strong scents, bright lights, and dramatic weather variations are a few examples of environmental elements that might cause persistent headaches.

Hormonal Changes: Chronic migraines may be exacerbated by hormonal fluctuations, which are especially common in women going through menopause, pregnancy, or the menstrual cycle.

Stress and worry: Chronic tension-type headaches are known to be triggered by emotional stress and worry.

Neurological Factors: Chronic headaches may be caused by abnormalities in the chemical or structural makeup of the brain.

Overuse of Medication: It is ironic that using painkillers and other drugs excessively might result in persistent daily headaches.

To sum up, persistent headaches are a complicated medical issue with many facets that need a thorough approach to diagnosis and treatment. Healthcare practitioners may customize treatment strategies to meet the unique requirements of patients with chronic headaches by knowing the different kinds, how they affect the quality of life, and the typical causes and triggers of these headaches. To reduce symptoms and enhance general well-being, a mix of medicines, lifestyle changes, and therapy treatments may be used.

CHAPTER TWO

Comprehending Prolonged Headaches

The complicated and often incapacitating nature of chronic headaches may have a major negative effect on a person's quality of life. It's critical to investigate the architecture of the head and neck, important structures and nerves, the relationship between the brain and skull, the neurological causes of headaches, and the function of neurotransmitters and pain pathways in order to build a simple solution strategy.

1. Anatomy Of The Head And Neck: The brain, muscles, blood vessels, nerves, and skull are among the many components that make up the head and neck. Knowing the anatomy is essential to understanding the possible causes of persistent headaches. Frequent causes include vascular problems, anomalies in the skull and surrounding tissues, or strain in the neck muscles.

2. Important Structures And Nerves:

A number of important structures and nerves are crucial in the development of headaches. For example, the trigeminal nerve plays a significant role in face feeling and may cause pain when it becomes inflamed. Tension-type headaches may also be caused by muscles in the neck and shoulders. Targeted treatments may be created by the identification of certain triggers associated with these structures.

3. Brain And Skull Interaction:

The brain is housed and protected inside the stiff structure that is the skull. Headaches may result from perturbations in the balance between the brain and the skull, such as elevated intracranial pressure or altered cerebral blood flow. Analyzing this relationship is essential to figuring out the underlying causes of persistent headaches and creating effective treatments.

4. Headache Basis:

An understanding of persistent headaches must take into account neurological variables. Headaches may arise and last for a long time due to anomalies in the central nervous system, changes in neurotransmitter levels, and changes in how the brain processes pain signals. Examining these neurological characteristics provides important information about possible therapeutic strategies.

5. Function Of Neurotransmitters:

Within the neurological system, neurotransmitters are essential chemical messengers that facilitate the transmission of impulses. Different kinds of headaches have been linked to imbalances in neurotransmitter levels, such as those of dopamine or serotonin. A simple solution strategy may include addressing these imbalances with medication, lifestyle changes, or other treatments.

6. Pain Channels: Managing persistent headaches requires an understanding of the channels by which pain signals move. For example, migraine headaches are related to the trigeminovascular system, but tension-type headaches may be related to the sensitivity of pain pathways in the muscles. Treatments that are specifically customized to address or prevent persistent headaches may be developed by focusing on certain pain pathways.

In summary, a thorough grasp of the anatomy of the head and neck, important structures and nerves, the relationship between the brain and skull, the neurological causes of headaches, the function of neurotransmitters, and the complexities of pain pathways is necessary for a simplified approach to treating chronic headaches. Healthcare providers may create individualized plans to manage and lessen the effects of chronic headaches on people's lives by methodically addressing these factors.

CHAPTER THREE

Recognizing Triggers

People may often lessen the frequency and severity of their headaches by being aware of and taking appropriate action against certain triggers. Let's examine the many categories of triggers, beginning with environmental ones.

Environmental Stressors:

1. Changes in the weather and atmosphere:

• For some people, abrupt variations in temperature, humidity, or barometric pressure might result in headaches.

• Observing relationships between headache incidence and weather patterns may be accomplished by keeping a headache journal.

2. Lighting Specifications:

• Bright or flickering lights, such as artificial and daylight illumination, may give people headaches, particularly those who are sensitive to light.

• Wearing a hat, sunglasses, or adjusting the lighting may all be beneficial.

3. Stress and Noise:

• Common triggers include loud sounds and high levels of stress.

• Headaches brought on by stress may be lessened by putting stress management strategies into practice, such as deep breathing or meditation.

Food Reactions:

1. Intolerances to Food:

• Certain foods, such as cheese, chocolate, and processed meats, may include ingredients that make certain people more prone to headaches.

• One useful tool for identifying individual causes is keeping a food diary and removing probable triggers.

2. Dehydration:

• Drinking too little water might cause dehydration, which is known to cause headaches.

• It's crucial to stay well hydrated throughout the day by consuming enough water.

3. Alcohol and Caffeine:

• Headaches may be brought on by abrupt changes in caffeine use, either from too much or withdrawal.

• Moderation is crucial when it comes to alcohol; red wine and certain spirits, in particular, are popular triggers.

Simplified Method Of Solving:

1. Determine and Monitor Triggers:

• Keep a headache journal to record possible triggers, such as the day, time, location, and food.

• Examine trends and connections between headache incidence and triggers.

2. Changes to the Environment:

• Modify your living or working space to reduce exposure to recognized triggers. This might include donning sunglasses, using noise-canceling headphones, or hanging blackout curtains.

3. Modifications to Diet:

• Gradually cut out possible dietary triggers and track changes in the frequency of headaches.

• Eat a balanced diet, making sure to eat at regular intervals and avoiding going extended periods without eating.

4. Handling Hydration:

• Make sure you drink enough water all day long.

• Restrict your intake of liquids that might cause dehydration, such as sugary or caffeinated drinks.

5. Handling Stress:

• Engage in stress-relieving activities such as yoga, meditation, or frequent exercise.

• Recognize and deal with the causes of ongoing stress in your personal and work life.

6. Consultation with Medical Specialists:

• See a medical expert, such as a neurologist or headache specialist, if identifying or managing triggers on your own proves to be difficult.

• Depending on the unique circumstances of each person, prescription drugs or preventative measures could be suggested.

A thorough awareness of dietary and environmental causes is essential to a streamlined approach to treating persistent headaches. People may manage and lessen the burden of chronic headaches in their everyday lives by methodically identifying and treating these causes. When necessary, consulting a specialist guarantees a customized and comprehensive approach to headache treatment.

CHAPTER FOUR

Lifestyle Changes For The Relief Of Chronic Headaches

The quality of life may be greatly affected by chronic headaches, but managing them effectively can be aided by making comprehensive lifestyle changes.

Among the many things to think about, practicing mindfulness and meditation, integrating stress-reduction methods, and relaxation exercises, and emphasizing good sleep hygiene are all very important. Let's explore each of these ideas in more detail:

1. Techniques For Stress Management:

Severe stress is often the cause of headaches. Using stress-reduction strategies helps ease tension and lessen headache frequency and severity. To encourage relaxation and stress alleviation, routines might include practices like progressive muscle relaxation, biofeedback, and deep breathing exercises.

2. Exercises For Relaxation:

Frequent relaxation techniques, like yoga or mild stretching, may alleviate tense muscles and enhance general well-being. Stress levels may also be lowered by partaking in enjoyable and calming activities like reading, listening to music, or spending time in nature.

3. Meditation & Mindfulness:

Techniques for mindfulness and meditation are effective ways to control persistent headaches. Through the promotion of a non-judgmental awareness of thoughts and sensations, these techniques support being in the present moment. Programs that teach mindfulness-based stress reduction (MBSR) and guided meditation sessions may be very helpful in improving mental health and decreasing the frequency of headaches.

4. Suitable Sleep Position:

Chronic headaches are often caused by little or poor-quality sleep. Developing routines that encourage sound sleep on a regular basis is part of practicing excellent sleep hygiene. This entails keeping a regular sleep schedule, abstaining from stimulants like coffee just before bed, and setting up a cozy sleeping space.

5. The Value Of Consistent Sleep:

In addition to being essential for general health, getting enough sleep each night may help manage persistent headaches. Developing a regular sleep schedule lowers the risk of headaches and improves the quality of sleep by regulating the body's internal clock. For optimum health, adults typically need 7-9 hours of sleep every night.

6. Establishing A Sleep-Friendly Ambience:

The quality of your sleep may be significantly affected by the surroundings in which you sleep. Make sure your bedroom is peaceful, quiet, and cold. To provide enough support, get pillows and a comfy mattress. Reduce the amount of time spent on electronics before bed to avoid blue light exposure, which may disrupt the body's normal circadian rhythm.

Including these lifestyle changes in your everyday routine will help you manage your persistent headaches more effectively. Maintaining consistency is crucial, and these strategies must be customized to each person's tastes and requirements.

Seeking advice from experts or healthcare professionals may provide tailored direction and assistance in putting these long-term alleviation options into practice. Remember that greater results in the management of persistent headaches might come from a comprehensive strategy that takes into account several facets of lifestyle.

CHAPTER FIVE

Dietary Adjustments As A Simplified Approach To Chronic Headaches

Many variables might contribute to chronic headaches, but one that people often ignore is their food. It may be possible to reduce or avoid persistent headaches by implementing certain dietary adjustments, especially by using an anti-inflammatory diet. Here is a thorough examination of this idea:

Anti-Inflammatory Food Plan:

Chronic headaches are among the many health problems that are assumed to be influenced by inflammation. Eating foods that assist in lowering inflammation in the body will help relieve headaches; this is the main goal of an anti-inflammatory diet.

Foods to Add:

Fruits and Vegetables: Packed with of anti-inflammatory nutrients, vitamins, and minerals, fruits and vegetables also reduce inflammation. Leafy greens, berries, and vibrant veggies are all great options.

Fatty Fish: Fish high in omega-3 fatty acids, such as sardines, salmon, and mackerel, have anti-inflammatory properties. These may be helpful in lowering the body's level of inflammation.

Nuts and Seeds: Rich in antioxidants and good fats, almonds, walnuts, and flaxseeds support an anti-inflammatory diet.

Whole Grains: Choose whole grains, such as oats, brown rice, and quinoa, since they include minerals and fiber that may help lower inflammation.

Herbs & Spices: Anti-inflammatory qualities may be found in turmeric, ginger, garlic, and cinnamon. You may reduce headaches and enhance taste by using them in your meals.

Foods to Steer Clear of:

Processed meals: Packed full of trans fats, preservatives, and additives, processed meals may aggravate inflammation. Steer clear of packaged meals, fizzy beverages, and snacks.

Added Sugars: Consuming too much sugar might cause inflammation. Reduce your intake of processed sweets, candies, and sugary drinks.

Refined carbs: Refined carbs, such as spaghetti and white bread, may raise blood sugar levels and cause inflammation. Instead, go for entire grains.

Red and Processed Meat: Reduce your consumption of these types of meats since they may aggravate inflammation. Choose lean protein sources such as fish, chicken, or plant-based substitutes.

Dairy Products: Dairy products may cause sensitivities in some people. Try cutting down on or giving up dairy to see if that affects how often you get headaches.

Strategies for Hydration:

Headaches are often brought on by dehydration. Staying well-hydrated is important for general health and may help avoid headaches.

Sufficient Intake of Water:

Maintain Consistent Hydration: Throughout the day, sip water at regular intervals. To guarantee convenient access to water, always have a bottle with you.

Keep an eye on the color of your urine. A light yellow tint indicates proper hydration. Amber or dark yellow hues might indicate dehydration.

Foods That Will Hydrate You: Add foods high in water content to your diet, such as celery, cucumbers, and watermelon.

Electrolyte Equilibrium:

Electrolytes are essential for preserving fluid equilibrium and averting dehydration.

Natural Electrolyte Sources: To maintain electrolyte balance, eat foods high in potassium (bananas, oranges, spinach) and magnesium (nuts, seeds, leafy greens).

Drinks Rich in Electrolytes: To replace the electrolytes lost via perspiration, try natural electrolyte beverages like coconut water.

In conclusion, a basic solution approach to treating persistent headaches must include eating an anti-inflammatory diet, drinking enough water, and preserving electrolyte balance. Even while these dietary adjustments may not be a panacea, they can be helpful in controlling and avoiding headaches, particularly when paired with other healthful lifestyle choices. It's best to get specialized advice from a healthcare expert before making any changes linked to your health.

CHAPTER SIX

Comprehensive Methods

Rather than only treating the symptoms, holistic methods to managing chronic headaches target the underlying causes and promote total well-being. Herbal treatments, yoga, and physical activity are three important holistic headache relief techniques. Acupuncture and acupuncture are also effective.

1. Both Acupressure And Acupuncture:

• Acupuncture: This ancient Chinese medical procedure involves the insertion of tiny needles into certain body locations in order to initiate the flow of energy and facilitate healing. Acupuncture may assist with persistent headaches by harmonizing the body's energy (Qi), enhancing blood circulation, and easing muscular tension. Acupuncture may be useful in lowering headache frequency and severity, according to research.

• Acupressure: Acupressure, like acupuncture, is a technique that involves pressing on certain body spots. Fingers, thumbs, or specialized tools may be used for this task. Acupressure has the potential to reduce stress, enhance blood circulation, and unlock stored energy. Acupressure points on the temples, the base of the skull, and between the eyebrows are especially used to relieve headaches.

2. Herbal Treatments:

• Butterbur: Research has been done on the possibility of butterbur extract lowering migraine frequency and intensity. It is said to offer muscle-relaxing and anti-inflammatory qualities. To prevent potentially dangerous ingredients present in raw or unprocessed butterbur, it is essential to utilize a standardized, purified version of butterbur.

• Feverfew: Traditionally, migraines and other types of headaches have been treated using the plant feverfew. It is believed to have vasodilatory and anti-inflammatory properties. According to some research, feverfew may lessen migraine frequency and severity.

• Peppermint Oil: Applying topically or inhaling peppermint oil might help relieve tension headaches. It may encourage relaxation and have a relaxing impact on the muscles. You may gently massage the temples with diluted peppermint oil.

3. Yoga In Conjunction With Physical Activity:

• Yoga: Yoga combines meditation, breath control, and physical postures. Regular yoga practice has been linked to a decrease in headache frequency and severity. Child's Pose and the Forward Fold are two yoga positions that may help reduce tension in the shoulders and neck, which are prominent areas of pain associated with headaches.

• Physical exercise: Engaging in regular physical exercise may enhance general health and lessen headache frequency. Exercise encourages the production of endorphins, which have anti-depressant and mood-enhancing properties. Exercises that burn calories quickly, like cycling, running, or fast walking, might be very helpful. But it's crucial to choose activities that don't cause or worsen headaches.

To sum up, a customized mix of these techniques is used in a holistic manner to treat persistent headaches. Before beginning any new therapy, it is essential to speak with medical specialists, particularly if the patient is currently receiving medical attention or is using prescription drugs.

CHAPTER SEVEN

Medication Administration

Effective drug management is essential for reducing symptoms and enhancing the quality of life for those who suffer from chronic headaches, which may be a difficult and incapacitating illness.

Many choices, from over-the-counter (OTC) medicines to prescription pharmaceuticals, may be taken into consideration when it comes to medication management. Now let's explore each category:

Beyond-the-Counter Selections:

1. Pain Management:

Acetaminophen (Tylenol): Often used to relieve mild to moderate pain, acetaminophen is typically well tolerated, yet taking too much of it might harm the liver.

Two nonsteroidal anti-inflammatory medicines (NSAIDs) that aid with pain relief and inflammation reduction are ibuprofen (Advil, Motrin) and naproxen (Aleve). Consultation with a healthcare provider is suggested since prolonged usage may result in negative effects.

2. Anti-Inflammatory Medication:

Aspirin: A traditional NSAID with anti-inflammatory qualities, aspirin helps relieve headaches. On the other hand, some people may have bleeding and stomach discomfort from it.

Prescription Drugs:

1. Medications for prevention:

Beta-Blockers: Originally created to treat cardiac problems, beta-blockers (such as propranolol) also work to prevent migraines by controlling blood flow. Cold extremities and tiredness are possible side effects.

Antidepressants (such as amitriptyline): Studies have shown that certain antidepressants may effectively prevent persistent headaches. They could have an impact on neurotransmitters that are involved in feeling pain.

2. Rescue Drugs:

Triptans, such as sumatriptan, are medications that are specifically made to treat migraines. They function by constricting blood vessels and lowering inflammation. When taken as soon as a migraine begins, it works best.

Preparations containing ergotamine: These narrow blood vessels and may be used to treat severe migraines. They are often used as a second-line therapy, however, and have greater adverse effects than triptans.

Things to Think About When Managing Medication:

1. Tailored Care Programs:

Customizing drug regimens for each patient is crucial. It is important to take into account variables such as the kind and frequency of headaches, general health, and any drug interactions.

2. Frequent Inspections and Modifications:

Managing chronic headaches often requires continuing observation. Frequent check-ins with medical professionals aid in evaluating the efficacy of the existing treatment plan and making any modifications.

3. Changes in Lifestyle:

The best results from medication management come when lifestyle modifications are included. The benefits of prescription drugs may be enhanced by stress reduction, consistent exercise, and getting enough sleep.

4. Expert Advice:

Consulting with medical experts is essential. Accurate diagnosis, side effect monitoring, and drug adjustments depending on patient response are all possible with their assistance.

5. Patient Instruction:

Better adherence to treatment programs is fostered when patients are empowered with information about their disease and the drugs provided to them.

To sum up, a thorough strategy for managing medicines for persistent headaches entails striking a careful balance between over-the-counter (OTC) products, prescription drugs, preventative measures, and rescue drugs.

A successful and comprehensive treatment strategy must include lifestyle changes, patient education, and regular contact with healthcare experts.

CHAPTER EIGHT

Getting Expert Assistance

Getting expert assistance is essential for treating persistent headaches because it enables people to obtain individualized treatment and direction. This is a thorough examination of getting medical attention for persistent headaches:

Experts In Headaches And Neurology:

Expertise in Diagnosis:

Medical professionals who specialize in problems of the nervous system, which includes the brain, are known as neurologists. Specialists in headaches are neurologists with extra training in headache care.

To find the underlying cause of persistent headaches, they may do comprehensive assessments that may include imaging scans, neurological exams, and other diagnostic procedures.

Tailored Care Programs:

Personalized treatment programs may be created by neurologists and headache experts depending on the particular kind and causes of headaches.

To successfully treat symptoms, this may include a mix of medication, lifestyle changes, and other therapies.

Continuous Observation:

Frequent consultations with neurologists enable ongoing evaluation of the treatment plan's efficacy.

To best control persistent headaches, modifications may be made as required.

Clinics For Pain Management:

Multidisciplinary Method:

A multidisciplinary approach is often used in pain treatment clinics, incorporating a range of medical specialists such as physicians, nurses, physical therapists, and psychologists.

This all-encompassing method tackles headaches as well as the psychological, emotional, and physical components of chronic pain.

Interventional Techniques:

Interventional therapies like Botox injections or nerve blocks are often provided by pain management clinics, and they may be useful in lowering the frequency and severity of headaches.

Instruction and Assistance:

Patients who visit pain treatment clinics are given instructions about coping mechanisms, lifestyle changes, and pain management practices.

People with chronic headaches might feel more connected to one another and understand one another via the support groups offered by these clinics.

Counselors And Therapists:

Psychological Assistance:

Counselors and therapists, particularly those with expertise in pain psychology, maybe a great resource for those who suffer from persistent headaches.

They support patients in investigating the psychological dimensions of pain, stress, and coping strategies.

Therapy based on cognitive behavior (CBT):

When it comes to treating persistent headaches, CBT is a very useful therapeutic method. It assists people in recognizing and altering harmful thinking patterns and actions that could be causing their headaches.

Handling Stress:

In order to assist people in better handling stress, which is a major cause of headaches, therapists may teach them mindfulness exercises, relaxation methods, and stress management strategies.

Biofeedback:

Biofeedback, which is often administered by therapists, teaches patients how to manage physiological processes like muscular tension that lead to pain. This may help in managing headaches.

Including Expert Assistance:

Cooperative Healthcare:

Collaboration between neurologists, pain management experts, and therapists is frequently necessary for successful headache care.

A more comprehensive and successful treatment strategy is facilitated by these specialists' regular contact and exchange of information.

Advocacy for Patients:

Seeking professional assistance entails speaking out for oneself as well as obtaining therapy. It is important for patients to actively share with their healthcare staff their symptoms, worries, and preferred course of therapy.

Extended-Term Management Approaches:

Experts can help people create long-term plans for dealing with persistent headaches, with a focus on self-care and sustainable lifestyle adjustments.

In summary, getting expert assistance for persistent headaches entails a thorough strategy that takes into account the lifestyle, psychological, and physical components of the ailment. Effective treatment of headaches requires open communication and collaborative care between the patient's healthcare team.

CHAPTER NINE
Alternative Medical Interventions

The quality of life may be greatly impacted by chronic headaches, but there are important treatment options available via alternative therapy. Three alternative methods stand out above the others: neuromodulation techniques, biofeedback, and chiropractic therapy.

Chiropractic Treatment:

Chiropractic treatment is centered on the interaction between the neurological system and the spine, acknowledging that subluxations, or misalignments in the spine, may impact general health, including headaches. The manual manipulation procedures used by chiropractors are intended to realign the spine and release stress.

Mechanism Of Action: The goals of chiropractic adjustments are to promote blood flow and nervous system performance. Chiropractic therapy may lessen headache frequency and severity by correcting misalignments.

Research Evidence: Although studies on the efficacy of chiropractic therapy for headaches are still being conducted, there is some indication that it may be helpful, particularly for migraines and tension-type headaches. Following chiropractic therapy, patients often report a reduction in the frequency and intensity of their headaches.

Taking Into Account: It's critical that those seeking chiropractic therapy choose a reputable and licensed chiropractor. Furthermore, a multidisciplinary strategy that incorporates various therapy modalities with chiropractic care may be advantageous.

Biofeedback: Biofeedback is a mind-body approach that teaches people how to manage physiological processes, such as muscular tension, heart rate, and skin temperature, with the use of electronic monitoring.

Mechanism Of Action: Real-time input about physiological reactions is provided by sensors affixed to the body during biofeedback sessions. Through behavioral tactics, relaxation techniques, and mental exercises, patients may learn to manage these reactions.

Research Verdict: Biofeedback has been shown to be effective in treating a variety of headache conditions, including migraines. Biofeedback helps people take charge of their physiological processes, which may lower headache frequency and severity and enhance general health.

Things to think about Since biofeedback is non-invasive and usually safe, it's a good choice for anyone looking for drug-free methods. For complete headache care, it is often used with other medicines.

Techniques For Neuromodulation: Applying electrical or magnetic stimulation to change nerve activity is known as neuromodulation. The goal of this method is to alter the aberrant brain activity linked to persistent headaches.

Neuromodulation Types:

The technique known as transcranial magnetic stimulation (TMS) involves stimulating brain nerve cells using magnetic fields.

Peripheral Nerve Stimulation (PNS): This modifies pain signals by placing electrodes in close proximity to peripheral nerves.

Empirical Support: Neuromodulation methods have shown potential in mitigating the frequency and intensity of persistent headaches, such as migraines. In particular, TMS has been researched for its potential to interfere with the aberrant brain activity linked to migraines.

Though neuromodulation is a potentially exciting topic, individual outcomes may differ. It is essential to speak with a healthcare provider to choose the best neuromodulation method and to make sure it is applied correctly.

Finally, non-traditional approaches to treating persistent headaches include chiropractic adjustments, biofeedback, and neuromodulation methods. To find the best, most individualized treatment for their particular disease, people must, nonetheless, collaborate closely with healthcare providers. The quality of life for those with chronic headaches may be improved and overall headache management can be strengthened by including these alternative treatments into a thorough treatment strategy.

Conclusion

In summary, it enables a simplified approach to treating chronic headaches

The quality of life may be greatly impacted by chronic headaches, but improved management and relief can be achieved by taking a straightforward solution approach.

In summary, it's critical to understand that treating chronic headaches involves a multimodal approach that takes into account a person's lifestyle, mental health, and general well-being.

Summary Of Crucial Techniques:

Finding Triggers: To start, identify the possible causes of persistent headaches. This might include monitoring trends associated with nutrition, sleep, stress, and environmental variables by maintaining an extensive headache journal.

Lifestyle Modifications: Even little adjustments to regular routines may have a big effect. Maintain a balanced diet, be hydrated, and follow a regular sleep pattern. Frequent exercise may also help avoid headaches, especially in milder forms like walking.

Stress Management Strategies: Stress and chronic headaches are often closely related. Include stress-reduction strategies in your everyday practice, such as deep breathing exercises, mindfulness, or meditation. These techniques may lessen headache frequency and severity as well as assist in controlling stress levels.

Hydration and Diet: Certain food components and dehydration may cause headaches. Drink plenty of water and think about eating a diet high in nutrient-dense foods. For some people, cutting down on alcohol and caffeine may be helpful.

Frequent Exercise: Studies have shown that regular exercise reduces the frequency and severity of headaches. Take part in frequent physical exercise that is appropriate for your level of fitness, such as yoga, brisk walks, or more strenuous activities. See a medical professional before beginning a new fitness regimen.

Medical Consultation: See a physician if your headaches don't go away. They may assist in determining any underlying medical concerns, propose additional therapies suited to your particular circumstances, or prescribe the proper drugs.

Motivation For Perseverance:

It may be difficult to treat persistent headaches, and results might not appear right away. Maintaining motivation and persistence is essential when putting these techniques into practice. Recognize that failures could happen, but that every attempt advances your knowledge of your triggers and useful coping mechanisms.

Celebrate your little progress along the road, and encourage yourself to do so. These successes—whether it's going a day without a headache or successfully forming a new habit—are crucial measures of development. Make sure you have a network of friends, family, or medical experts at your side who can provide support and direction.

Recall that each person's path to improved headache control is unique, and that perseverance is essential. Remain dedicated to the process, practice self-compassion, and recognize that little steps toward progress are worthwhile ones.

Giving Readers The Tools To Take Charge:

The key to treating persistent headaches is empowerment. You recover control over your life by realizing what's causing your headaches and taking proactive steps to make good adjustments. The following are essential strategies for self-empowerment:

Education: Get to know the causes, symptoms, and practical treatment techniques of the particular kind of headaches you have. Your ability to make educated choices and work well with healthcare providers is enhanced by knowledge.

Self-Advocacy: Participate actively in your medical treatment. Openly explore treatment alternatives, share your experiences, and engage in dialogue with your healthcare practitioner. Speak out for your preferences and requirements to guarantee a tailored and successful strategy.

Mind-Body Connection: Acknowledge the relationship between mental and physical health. Techniques like mindfulness, meditation, and cognitive-behavioral therapy may help you become more adept at controlling stress and how it affects your headaches.

Adaptability: Recognize that treating persistent headaches requires constant attention. Be prepared to modify your tactics to suit your needs as they arise. Review often and modify your strategy as necessary.

Join support groups to meet others who also suffer from persistent headaches. Exchange knowledge, perspectives, and coping mechanisms. Creating a support system may be a great way to get both helpful guidance and emotional support.

Finally, a one-size-fits-all strategy for treating persistent headaches is not appropriate for all cases. It is a customized, all-encompassing approach that includes medication, stress reduction techniques, and lifestyle adjustments. Through the provision of essential methods, motivation to persevere, and empowerment to assume responsibility, people may start a voyage towards enhanced headache management and a higher quality of life.

THE END